Cut out sugar:

Steps to identify hidden sweets, reduce cravings, and overcome addiction.

By

Mark L. White

publisher's consent must be gained. Therefore, the contents within can neither be electronically, transferred, nor kept in a database. Neither in part nor full can the document be copied, scanned, fixed or retained without approval from the publisher or creator.

Table of contents

INTRODUCTION

Sugar is a kind of carbohydrate. The body converts all carbs into sugar. Sugars are classified into many categories based on their molecular structure. Monosaccharides are the simplest kind of sugar since they only contain one sugar molecule. They include: Milk includes glucose and galactose, whereas fruits often contain fructose. Disaccharides or polysaccharides are sugars containing two or more molecules. This includes: Sucrose is a commonly used table sugar, while lactose is found in milk and dairy products.

The body converts carbs to glucose, which enters the circulation and serves as a source of energy. Some sugars, including glucose, fructose, and lactose, exist naturally in foods and beverages.

Added sugars are any sugars in foods that are not naturally occurring, such as sugar in baked goods. Foods and beverages may also include highly processed sugars, such as high fructose corn syrup.

Sugars appear on food and drink labels, therefore those who want to restrict their sugar intake can search for the following on ingredient lists:

Raw sugar, corn sweetener, or syrup

High fructose corn syrup.

The body has a natural feedback system that causes high glucose levels to enhance insulin production and low levels to reduce this hormone. To function effectively, the body requires adequate insulin levels. Diabetes can occur when there is insufficient insulin or when it no longer acts correctly. Therefore, inside this book, you will learn the Steps to identify hidden sweets, reduce cravings, and overcome addiction for life, sit, relax and stay tuned for these life changing steps.

CHAPTER 1

Sugar can lead to overeating and harm your health.

Sugar is fine for you in limited quantities, however, an excessive amount can prompt weight gain, skin breakout, and type 2 diabetes, and can expand your gamble of a few serious clinical conditions. From marinara sauce to peanut butter, added sugar can be tracked down in even the most surprising items. Many individuals depend on speedy, handled food sources for dinners and tidbits. Since these items frequently contain added sugar, it make up a huge extent of their everyday calorie consumption. An estimated 17 teaspoons of added sugar are consumed daily by the typical adult in the United States. That records for 14% of complete calorie consumption in grown-ups following a 2,000-calorie diet. Specialists accept that sugar utilization is a significant reason for weight and numerous constant illnesses, like sort 2 diabetes.

That is the reason dietary rules propose restricting calories from added sugar to under 10% each day.

1. It Might Make You Gain Weight;

Obesity rates are increasing around the world, and proof recommends that additional sugar — frequently from sugar-sweetened drinks — is a significant supporter of stoutness. Sugar-sweetened drinks like soft drinks, juices, and sweet teas are stacked with fructose, a kind of straightforward sugar. Devouring fructose expands your yearning and craving for food more than glucose, the primary kind of sugar tracked down in bland food sources. Additionally, animal research indicates that excessive fructose intake may result in resistance to leptin, an essential hormone that controls hunger and signals the body to stop eating. All in all, sweet drinks don't check your craving, making it simple to polish off countless fluid calories rapidly. This can prompt weight gain. Research shows that consuming sweet refreshments is related to weight gain and expanded chance of type 2 diabetes.

Likewise, drinking a ton of sugar-sweetened refreshments is connected to an expanded measure of instinctive fat, a sort of profound stomach fat related to conditions like diabetes and coronary illness.

2. Unhealthy Sugar Consumption may put your Heart Health at Risk:

High sugar has been related to an expanded gamble of numerous sicknesses, including coronary illness, the main source of death around the world. Proof recommends that high-sugar diets can prompt heftiness and aggravation as well as high fatty oils, glucose, and circulatory strain levels —

which are all chance elements for coronary illness. Furthermore, polishing off an excess of sugar, particularly from sugar-sweetened drinks, has been connected to atherosclerosis, an illness described by greasy, supply routes stopping up deposits. A concentrate on north of 25,877 grown-ups found that people who drank more added sugar had a more serious gamble of creating coronary illness and coronary complexities

contrasted with people who drank less added sugar Not in the least does expanded sugar consumption increment cardiovascular gamble, however it can likewise build

hazard of stroke. Only one 12-ounce (473-ml) container of pop contains 39 grams of sugar, which compares to 8% of your everyday calorie utilization, given a 2,000-calorie diet. This implies that one sweet beverage daily can bring you near the suggested day as far as possible for added sugar.

3. Connected to Skin Inflammation :
Acne development has been linked to a diet high in refined carbohydrates, such as sugary foods and beverages. Food sources with a higher glycemic record, for example, handled desserts, raise your glucose more quickly than food sources with a lower glycemic index. Consuming sweet food sources can cause a spike in glucose and insulin levels, prompting expanded androgen discharge, oil creation, and irritation — all of which assume a skin part break-out improvement. Proof has shown that low-glycemic counts of calories are related to a diminished skin inflammation risk, while high-glycemic eats less are connected to a higher skin inflammation risk.

Furthermore, numerous populace studies have shown that rustic networks that eat conventional, non-handled food sources have a lot of lower paces of skin break out contrasted with more metropolitan, major league salary regions where handled food is important for a standard eating routine. These discoveries harmonize with the hypothesis that slim in handled, sugar-loaded food varieties add to the improvement of skin breakout.

4. Unhealthy Sugar Consumption may put you at Risk of Developing Type 2 Diabetes:

Diabetes is one of the leading causes of death and shorter life expectancy. Over the past 30 years, its prevalence has more than doubled, and projections indicate that its burden will continue to rise. "Unhealthy sugar consumption is strongly linked to an increased risk of developing diabetes. Consuming too much sugar can lead to weight gain, which is one of the leading risk factors for type 2 diabetes. In addition, high sugar intake can cause insulin resistance, which can lead to the development of diabetes over time. Therefore, it's important to limit sugar intake to help reduce the risk of developing diabetes."

Consuming a lot of sugar can make you more likely to get diabetes by making you gain weight and have more fat in your body, both of which are risk factors for diabetes. Weight, which is much of the time brought about by inordinate sugar utilization, is viewed as the most grounded risk factor for diabetes. Furthermore, drawn-out high-sugar utilization drives protection from insulin, a chemical created by the pancreas that manages glucose levels. Insulin obstruction causes glucose levels to rise and unequivocally expands your gamble of diabetes.

5. It May Build Your Gamble of Disease:

Eating over-the-top measures of sugar might expand your gamble of fostering specific malignant growths. First, eating a diet high in sugary foods and drinks can make you overweight, which raises your cancer risk significantly. Additionally, counting calories high in sugar increment aggravation in your body and may cause insulin obstruction, the two of which increment disease risk. A precise survey examining 37 planned partner investigations discovered that in two of five examinations
on added sugar, a 60% - 95% expanded disease risk was seen with higher sugar admissions.

6. It Might Make You More Likely to Get Depressed:
While a sound eating routine can assist with working on your temperament, an eating regimen high in added sugar and handled food sources might add to changes in mindset and feelings. You

might even be more likely to experience depression as a result of it. High sugar utilization has been connected to mental weaknesses, memory issues, and profound problems like tension and wretchedness. Scientists trust that constant fundamental irritation, insulin obstruction, and an upset dopaminergic reward flagging framework — which can all be brought about by expanded sugar utilization — may add to sugar's impeding effect on emotional wellness. A review following 8,000 individuals showed that men who consumed 67 grams or a greater amount of sugar each day were 23% more bound to foster discouragement than men who ate under 40 grams each day.

7. Unhealthy sugar consumption may accelerate the aging process of your skin:

Wrinkles are a common visible sign of skin aging. Regardless of your health, they will show up eventually. However, poor eating can exacerbate wrinkles and accelerate skin aging. In your body, reactions between sugar and protein result in the formation of compounds known as advanced glycation end products (AGEs). Sugars have been implicated as a key contributor to skin aging. Consuming an eating regimen high in refined carbs and sugar prompts the development of AGEs, which might make your skin age rashly. AGEs harm collagen and elastin, which are proteins that help the skin stretch and keep its young appearance. When collagen and elastin become harmed, the skin loses its immovability and starts to droop.

8. It Can Prompt Fatty Liver:

A high admission of fructose has been reliably connected to an expanded gamble of greasy liver. Fructose is a typical sort of sugar, with one significant source being high fructose corn syrup

(HFCS) used to improve pop, treats, prepared products, oats, and the sky is the limit
from there. Fructose in contrast to glucose and other types of sugar, which are absorbed by a large number of cells throughout the body, is almost entirely broken down by the liver. In the liver, fructose is changed over into energy or put away as glycogen. However, the liver can unfortunately store a limited amount a lot of glycogen before abundance sums are transformed into fat. Large measures of added sugar as fructose overburden your liver, prompting nonalcoholic fatty liver illness (NAFLD), a condition described by unnecessary fat development in the liver.

CHAPTER 2
Sugar Hidden from View

Most Americans eat an excessive amount of sugar. The issue is that many individuals don't know about it. That is because sugar remains unnoticed without really having to try numerous food sources you eat every day. From bread to store meat, sugar is all over.

You ought to check the fixings arrangements of the food sources you purchase to guarantee you're not getting an excess of added sugar in your eating routine, however, sugar additionally has a few names you may not naturally perceive and in this manner keep away from. Added sugar is stowing away in 74% of bundled food varieties. We will generally believe that additional sugar is fundamentally found in sweets like treats and cakes, but at the same time, it's tracked down in numerous flavorful food sources, for example, bread and pasta sauce. Furthermore, a few food varieties advanced as "regular" or "solid" are weighed down with added sugars, intensifying the disarray.

Producers add sugar to 74% of packaged food sources sold in grocery stores. Along these lines, regardless of whether you skip dessert, you might in any case be consuming more added sugar than is suggested.

How can I tell if I'm eating sugar added to my food?

Added sugar is concealed in food varieties that large numbers of us consider sound, similar to yogurt and energy bars. It is additionally added to flavorful food varieties, for example, ketchup, bread, salad dressing, and pasta sauce.

The U.S. Food and Medication Organization (FDA) requires food makers to list all fixings in their food sources.

However, added sugar comes in many structures - which is the reason it's so elusive on the fixings mark. There are something like 61 distinct names for sugar recorded on food marks. While item names list complete sugar content, producers are not expected to say whether that product has incorporated added sugar, which makes it hard to tell the amount of the outcomes from added sugar and how much is normally happening in fixings like

natural products or milk. That makes it truly challenging to represent how much-added sugar we're consuming.

How much sugar is all right?

Day to day Added Sugar Cutoff points women: 6 tsp. (25g) Men: 9 tsp. (38g) children: 3-6 tsp. (12-25g). Dissimilar to salt and fats that are added to food varieties, nourishment marks don't give you an everyday reference an incentive for added sugar.

In any case, the American Heart Association(AHA) suggests something like 9 teaspoons (38 grams) of added sugar each day for men and 6 teaspoons (25 grams) for women. The AHA limits for children vary depending on their age and caloric needs, but range between 3-6 teaspoons (12 - 25 grams) each day.

Indeed "sound" food sources can be high in sugar

With upwards of 11 teaspoons (46.2 grams) of added sugar in some 12-oz. soft drinks, a solitary serving surpasses the AHA proposal for men and is about two times the remittance for ladies and children. However, beverages and sweet baked goods contain sugar as well.

Here are a few solid-looking things you could find in the store that likewise have high sugar contents:

- One driving brand of yogurt contains 7 teaspoons (29 grams) of sugar per serving.

- A morning meal bar made with "genuine natural product" and "entire grains" records 15 grams of sugar.

- A morning meal bar made with "genuine natural product" and "entire grains" records 15 grams of sugar.

- A product containing cranberry/pomegranate juice has 30 grams of added sugar per 8-ounce serving, despite advertising "no high-fructose corn syrup" and "100% Vitamin C." A portion of the sugar is normally happening, however some of it has been added.

CHAPTER 3

Addiction to sugar

As indicated by a recent report, "discontinuous admittance to sugar can prompt way of behaving and neurochemical changes that look like the impacts of a substance of misuse."

Any substance that we use for joy can be an addiction — this incorporates sugar. Research shows that our minds are designed for joy, and sugar works similarly to numerous habit-forming drugs in that it influences the cerebrum's limbic framework, the piece of the mind that is related to profound control.

Mind checks show that irregular sugar utilization influences the cerebrum similar to specific medications, so the following time you hunger for something sweet, it very well might be something other than a sweet tooth: it very well may be an expansion you want to address. The diary Neuroscience and Biobehavioral Surveys found that sugar meets the rules for a substance of misuse, and the people who gorge on it very well may be addicted.

Food addiction is conceivable since cerebrum pathways have advanced to answer normal prizes and in this way become actuated by habit-forming drugs. A review from Science Direct reasoned that sugar discharges narcotics, and dopamine, hence, could have this habit-forming potential. There were four parts of sugar dependence broke down, including:

- Binging,
- Withdrawal
- Craving
- Cross-sensitization

These parts were exhibited typically with sugar gorging being the reinforcer, and are connected with neurochemical changes in the mind that additionally happen with habit-forming drugs. In specific situations, rodents can become dependent on sugar, which might mean a few human circumstances that might incorporate dietary problems and obesity.

Sugar Addiction Manifestations

The manifestation of sugar addiction can differ from one individual to another, yet a few normal signs and side effects might include:

- Powerful desires for sweet food varieties or drinks, particularly in the wake of polishing off them.
- Trouble controlling or restricting the utilization of sweet food sources. Diligent craving for sweet preferences and the requirement for progressively bigger measures of sugar to encounter fulfillment.

- Withdrawal-like side effects while endeavoring to scale back or quit sugar, for example, peevishness, mindset swings, cerebral pains, or exhaustion.
- Proceeded with the utilization of sweet food varieties regardless of unfortunate results on actual well-being or in general prosperity.
- A constant desire for the next sugar fix and a preoccupation with thoughts of sugary foods.
- Trouble keeping a reasonable and sound eating routine because of the overwhelming impact of sugar desires.
- Expanded resistance to sugar, prompting the requirement for higher amounts or more extreme flavors to encounter a similar degree of fulfillment.

Note that sugar addiction isn't perceived as a conventional determination in clinical or mental writing. However, many people struggle to control their sugar intake and experience intense cravings, both of which can have a significant negative impact on their overall health and well-being.

CHAPTER 4

Breaking your Dependence on Sugar

The normal insight goes: *move more, eat less* . Imagine if it were that easy! The fact of the matter is that the food industry has managed to control not only our taste buds but also the chemicals and hormones in our brains.

We fault ourselves for consuming an excessive amount of sugar. Yet, even the individuals who are aware of how the chemicals and synapses that fuel sugar desires work struggle with bridling the devices to battle them when such countless dollars are channeled into driving this organic problem.

The possibility of surrendering sugar altogether can appear to be overwhelming, yet it's 100% conceivable to figure out how to scale back and release sugar's hold on everything you might do.

Here are demonstrated strategies to assist you with breaking your sugar compulsion for good.

- **Sugar substitutes are not escaped prison-free cards**

While sugar substitutes can be advantageous and safe, they can likewise screw with your digestion and fuel hunger. "Substitutes can assist with people who are eating less junk food, who experience the ill effects of diabetes (since a few counterfeit sugars don't cause a sharp spike in glucose), and the people who are stressed over pits and tooth rot brought about by sugar,".

Very much like with standard white sugar, it underlines that it's vital to devour fake sugars with some restraint and get the greater part of your calories from entire food varieties. Yet, how to do this? Peruse on for master-endorsed strategies for eating (and drinking) less sugar.

"Healthy" Foods Have A Lot More Sugar Than You Think

- **Get more rest.**

Individuals don't understand it, however not resting well can influence your sugar desires. Studies have shown that unfortunate rest prompts more profound desires for desserts. On top of rolling out a few dietary improvements, it's critical to take a gander at your rest designs. To assist with cravings, go for the nine hours of rest/sleep each night.

- **Know the distinction between cravings and hunger.**

Customarily when we believe we're eager, we're simply having a craving.

What's the distinction? Next time you need to go after that chocolate cake, ask yourself: assuming the main thing I needed to eat right presently was an apple, could I eat it? If the response is "no," you probably have a craving rather than being hungry.

At the point when you're eager, what you're willing to eat is adaptable, while you have a desire, it's not. The following time you reply "no" to that inquiry, require 20 minutes before you follow up on it. Frequently you'll find that the desire disappears; on the off chance that it doesn't then permit yourself to enjoy it carefully.

"You can likewise attempt to supplant that cravings with a solid substitute,"

E.g: Whenever I experience a desire, I'll either take a walk or taste shining water. I view that as if I don't follow up on my underlying craving and permit an opportunity to pass, my desire will normally scatter all alone.

- **Add a protein to a carb-rich breakfast.**

A review that saw X-ray outputs of individuals having a high-protein breakfast found diminished action in the locales of the mind related with desires. Have a go at adding protein to your morning meal and check whether it assists you with eliminating sugar later in the day

On the off chance that you're eating a bagel or toast, incorporate some smoked salmon to get the advantages of protein.

- **Make structure.**

Think not much about killing sugar, and on second thought reevaluate it as adding a greater amount of the great stuff to your eating routine. Mean to reliably fill your plate with protein, solid fat, and high-fiber carbs like non-boring vegetables.

- **Go for segment/portion control.**

Since sugar fixation is organic — not profound with no guarantees so frequently thought — this probably won't work for everybody. Many individuals can't live by

"three-chomp rules," yet that has only good intentions in attempting.

One way to achieve this is to purchase higher-sugar foods in single-serving sizes, which can help you control your portions at mealtime. For example, If you don't have beyond four Oreos at home, you can't eat multiple Oreos.

- **Remove sugar in food sources that aren't sweet.**

If you can't surrender your frozen yogurt and chocolate, attempt to dispense with ketchup and salsa. "It's important to be

aware that sugar is found in many ingredients and sauces, and it's not only present in desserts or sweet foods." It can likewise be found in certain dinners, for example, sushi rice and polenta."
Producers add sugar to 74 percent of bundled food varieties! "If you look closely at the ingredient labels of processed foods, you'll find sugar hiding everywhere — even in foods that are marketed as healthy, like breakfast bars that claim to contain fruit and whole grains. These foods can often contain 15 grams or more of added sugar.
It's important to be aware of how much sugar you're consuming, as it can have negative effects on your health."Unknowingly, sugar cravings are conditioned in adults, children, toddlers, and even infants.

- **Drink a lot of water**

There's an explanation that a doctor finds that he can extinguish a portion of his yearning for sweet food varieties with water — frequently individuals mistake thirst for hunger. "It's an incredible trade for different beverages and it assists with sensations of completion, which might forestall accidental eating of sweet food varieties.

In one review, individuals who expanded their everyday water admission diminished their day-to-day sugar consumption." Along these lines, important improved drinks, similar to pop, lemonade, and sports drinks, are the main wellspring of added sugar in our weight control plans. If you find this difficult, try starting by reducing the amount you drink.

For example, *you could have a soda every other day instead of every day, on the off chance that you experience difficulty doing this, you can begin by cutting the sum you drink, for example, by having a soft drink every day rather than each day. Then, keep cutting back on how much you drink each week until you stop the habit."*

CHAPTER 5

Overcoming Obstacles like Withdrawal, Cravings, and Triggers .

Taking Care of Sugar-Related Obstacles:

What Causes Sugar Desires?

Sugar is profoundly imbued in our food framework and our day-to-day routines. Some of the time it seems like we must choose the option to eat it, considering the number of food varieties, refreshments, and nibble things it's additional to. On the other hand, you might desire desserts more than you'd like. How about we take a gander at a portion of the top reasons you could desire sugar?

What Is Sugar Withdrawal?

Might You at any point Rework Your Desires?

While there's something to be said about retraining your sense of taste, opposing all of your sugar desires at the same time might advance a greater amount of them — temporarily.

There is evidence to suggest that learning to resist sugar cravings can help recondition your sugary habits in the long run.

Meanwhile, hammering out a fair compromise that permits a few desserts as a component of a general supplement-rich eating regimen might assist with making progress simpler. All things considered, food wasn't simply intended to feed the body; it was likewise intended to give us pleasure. On the off chance that we can find a sound method for doing that, there ought not to be any disgrace or culpability in enjoying the food sources we appreciate.

Instructions to Stop Sugar Desires

Tips To Utilize at present

It may take some time to reduce and eventually eliminate sugar cravings. Here are ways to start retraining your sense of taste and overhauling your cerebrum/brain.

Try not to go "pure and simple": While this approach might work for some, permit yourself to partake in a few little treats as opposed to eliminating all that you need at the same time. Disposing of sugar from your eating routine "pure and simple" may set off sugar withdrawal.

Join food sources: Here and there, mixes can offer good food varieties with a touch of pleasantness that can relieve a desire. For example, have a go at plunging apples or strawberries in chocolate or eating a modest bunch of pecans with chocolate chips and raisins.

Get your brain off it: At times, we hunger for sugar out of sheer fatigue. Go for a speedy stroll or exercise and perceive how you feel when you return.

Drink enough water: We frequently confuse our requirement for hydration with a longing to eat. Take a stab at drinking water to check whether it decreases your sugar cravings.

Rest all things being equal: Feeling drained and apathetic? This can be an ideal time for sugar cravings to emerge. All things considered lay down for a midday rest and re-energize.

Make a trade: Instead of your go-to sweet treat, have a go at something different that can assist with fulfilling a craving. For example, attempt a better other option, similar to a natural product, dim chocolate, or custom-made trail blend.

Eat routinely: Skipping dinners can set you up for additional desires as your body goes into endurance mode. Maintaining a regular diet can help you remain satisfied.

Instructions to Diminish Sugar Consumption: *Long-term strategies for curbing sugar cravings*

Another methodology is to track down ways of halting sugar desires before they start. These could include;

Avoid artificial sugars: Resting on super sweet fake sugars might demolish desires for genuine sugar.

Reward yourself: Pick a non-food thing as opposed to compensating yourself with sweet treats when you arrive at specific achievements in your day-to-day existence.

For example, you could take yourself to the films or purchase a couple of earphones you've been needing. This can assist with retraining your mind to anticipate these things versus sugar.

Slow down because diet culture can be noisy and hard to focus on. Attempt to rehearse care, zeroing in on the thing you're eating and paying attention to your own body however much as could reasonably be expected.

Get help: It's hard to break bad habits, especially on our own. If you live with somebody or have a companion who battles with comparable sugar desires, take on this change together. Friends who hold you accountable can be very helpful in your development.

Attempt numerous procedures: There's seldom a convenient solution for anything we need to change. Something might work for a brief period however at that point ends up being fruitless.

Make it a point to turn and have a go at something new or a blend of approaches until you track down something that works for you.

Back off of yourself: Making heads or tails of sugar desires is difficult. Show restraint toward yourself as you see which approaches work — and which don't. Sugar cravings are very common and result from a variety of factors, so try not to feel shame or guilt about them.

CHAPTER 6

The most Effective Method to Deal with the Stressors, Mishaps, and Prevailing difficulty.

How does Stress Reduction Work?

It might appear as though you have no control over stress. Be that as it may, you have much surprising control. Assuming you're living with elevated degrees of stress, you're jeopardizing your whole prosperity.

Stress unleashes destruction on your close-to-home balance, as well as your general physical and emotional well-being.

It limits your capacity to think obviously, capability successfully, and appreciate life. You can be happier, healthier, and more productive if you can break the hold that stress has on your life through effective stress management. That is the reason it's critical to analyze and figure out what turns out best for you.

The accompanying stress and the executive's tips can assist you with doing that.

Tip 1: **Recognize the wellsprings of stress in your life**

Finding the causes of your stress in your life is the first step in stress management. This isn't quite as direct as it sounds. It is simple to identify major stressors like moving, going through a divorce, or changing jobs, but it can be more difficult to identify the causes of chronic stress.

It's quite barely noticeable how your contemplations, sentiments, and ways of behaving add to your regular feelings of anxiety. Without a doubt, you might realize that you're continually stressed over work cutoff times, yet perhaps it's your hesitation, as opposed to the genuine work requests, that is causing the pressure. To recognize what's sincerely worrying you, take a gander at your propensities, disposition, and excuse.

Even though you can't remember the last time you took a break, do you try to deflect stress by saying, "I just have a million things going on right now"?

Do you characterize pressure as an essential piece of your work or home life ("Things are consistently insane around here") or as a piece of your character ("I have a ton of apprehensive energy, there's nothing more to it")?

Do you view your stress as completely normal and unexceptional, or do you attribute it to other people or unforeseen occurrences? Until you acknowledge liability regarding the job you play in making or keeping up with it, your anxiety will stay unchangeable as far as you might be concerned.

Begin a stress diary

A stress diary can assist you with distinguishing the customary stressors in your day-to-day existence and how you manage them. Each time you feel worried, make a note of it in your diary or utilize a pressure tracker on your telephone. Keeping an everyday log will empower you to see examples and normal subjects. Take down:

- What caused your stress (make speculation if you're uncertain)?

- How you felt emotionally and physically.
- How you acted accordingly.
- How you cheered yourself up.

Tip 2: **Cut out unfortunate approaches to managing stress**

A considerable lot of us feel so worried, we resort to undesirable and inefficient ways of adapting. While many of these harmful tactics may temporarily lessen stress, in the long run, they do more harm:

- Smoking, drinking excessively or utilizing medications to unwind.
- Bingeing on junk or comfort food.
- Daydreaming for quite a long time before the television or telephone.
- Withdrawing from social activities and friends and family.
- Resting excessively.
- Topping off each moment of the day to try not to deal with issues.
- Procrastinating.

- Taking out your weight on others (erupting, unexpected eruptions of fury, actual brutality).

It's time to find healthier ways to cope with stress that leave you feeling calm and in control if they aren't improving your mental and physical health.

***Tip 3:* Practice Stress Management's four A's.**

While your nervous system will automatically respond to stress, certain stressors, such as the commute to work, a meeting with your boss, or family gatherings, can be anticipated. While dealing with such unsurprising stressors, you can either change what is happening or change your response.

While choosing which choice to make in some random situation, it's useful to consider the four A's: Avoid (stay away from), Alter (modify), Adjust, or Accept.

- **Avoid/stay away from unnecessary stress**

Not beneficial to keep away from a distressing circumstance should be tended to, however, you might be shocked by the number of stressors in your day-to-day existence that you can wipe out.

Figure out how to say "no": Know your cutoff points and stick to them. Taking on more than you can handle, whether in your personal or professional life, is a surefire way to cause stress.

Stay away from individuals who worry you: Assuming somebody reliably causes pressure in your life, limit how much time you spend with that individual, or terminate the friendship.

Take charge of your surroundings: Assuming the nightly news makes you restless, switch off the television. Online grocery shopping is a better option if going to the market is a chore you don't like.

Stay away from controversial points: Assuming you lash out over religion or governmental issues, cross them off your discussion list. Assuming you more than once quarrel over a similar subject with similar individuals, quit bringing it up or pardon yourself when it's the subject of conversation.

Pare down your daily agenda: Examine your daily routine, responsibilities, and schedule. On the off chance that you have a lot for you to handle, recognize the "shoulds" and the "musts. Prioritize the essential tasks and move the less important ones to the bottom of your to-do list — or simply delete them from your list entirely.

Sometimes we get bogged down by a long list of things to do, but when we think about it, some of those tasks aren't essential. Focusing on the important ones can help you feel less overwhelmed and more productive."

- **Alter what is going on**

If you can't keep away from a distressing circumstance, attempt to change it. Frequently, this includes altering how you convey and work in your day-to-day routine.

Express your sentiments as opposed to suppressing them. Assuming a person or thing is irritating you, impart your interests openly and consciously. If you don't voice your sentiments, disdain will assemble and the pressure will increase. Split the difference.

At the point when you request that somebody change their way of behaving, do likewise. If you both twist a bit, you'll have a decent possibility of tracking down a blissful center ground. Be more decisive.

Try not to assume a lower priority in your own life. Manage issues head-on, giving you all to expect and forestall them. Assuming you have a test to read up for and your loquacious flatmate just returned home, say front and center that you just have five minutes to talk.

Track down balance. Burnout is a recipe for doing nothing but work. Attempt to track down harmony among work and everyday life, social exercises and single pursuits, day-to-day obligations, and free time.

- **Adapt to the Stressors**

Change yourself if you are unable to change the stressor. By altering your expectations and attitude, you can adjust to stressful situations and regain control.

Reevaluate issues. Attempt to see distressing circumstances from a more inspirational outlook. Instead of seething about a gridlock, view it as a potential chance to stop and refocus, pay attention to your #1 radio broadcast, or partake in some alone time.

Check the higher perspective out.

Ask yourself how significant it will be in the grand scheme of things. Sometimes, things that seem like a big deal at the moment are not that important in the long run.

A different perspective can help you overcome the challenge and move on.". Will it matter in a month? A year? Is it truly worth blowing up finished? Assuming that the response is no, center your significant investment somewhere else.

Change your norms. Compulsiveness is a significant wellspring of avoidable pressure. Quit getting yourself positioned for disappointment by requesting flawlessness. Set sensible guidelines for yourself and others, and figure out how to be alright with "sufficient." Practice appreciation.

At the point when stress is getting you down, pause for a minute to ponder everything you value in your life, including your positive characteristics and gifts. You can use this straightforward strategy to keep things in perspective.

- **Accept the things you can't change**

Some sources of stress are unavoidable. You can't forestall or change stressors, for example, the passing of a loved one, a difficult disease, or a public downturn. Accepting things as they are is the best way to deal with stress in these situations. Acknowledgment might be troublesome, yet over the long haul, it's simpler than coming down on a circumstance you can't change.

Try not to attempt to control the wild. Numerous things in life are unchangeable as far as we might be concerned, especially the way of behave of others. As opposed to worrying over them, center around the things you have some control over like the way you decide to respond to issues.

Search for the potential gain.
While confronting significant difficulties, attempt to view them as any open doors for self-improvement. If your own unfortunate decisions added to an unpleasant circumstance, ponder them and gain from your slip-ups.

Figure out how to excuse. Accepting this fact can help you develop more compassion and understanding for others, and it can help you move past disappointment and frustration."Let go of your resentment and anger. Free yourself from negative energy by excusing and continuing.

Express your emotions. Even if there is nothing you can do to alleviate the stress, expressing your feelings can be very therapeutic. Converse with a confided-in companion or make a meeting with a specialist.

***Tip 4:* Get Rolling at the Point**

When you're anxious, the last thing you presumably want to do is get up and work out. However, actual work is a tremendous pressure reliever — and you don't need to be a competitor or go through hours in an exercise center to encounter the advantages. Exercise can help you feel better by releasing endorphins and providing a helpful distraction from your day-to-day worries. While you'll get the most advantage from consistently practicing for 30 minutes or more, it's OK to develop your wellness level slowly. Indeed, even tiny exercises can accumulate throughout the day. "The first step is to take action.

Here are simple methods for integrating exercise into your day-to-day plan:

- Put on some music and dance around.
- Take your canine for a walk.
- Walk or cycle to the supermarket.

- Utilize the steps at home or work as opposed to a lift.
- Leave your vehicle in the farthest spot in the part and walk the remainder of the way.
- As you exercise, encourage one another by joining forces with a workout partner.
- Play an activity-based video game or ping pong with your kids.
- Manage stress with careful cadenced activity.

While pretty much any type of actual work can assist with consuming with smoldering heat pressure and stress, musical exercises are particularly successful.

Great decisions incorporate strolling, running, swimming,

moving, cycling, kendo, and vigorous exercise. Be that as it may, anything you pick, ensure it's something you appreciate so you're bound to stay with it. While you're working out, put forth a cognizant attempt to focus on your body and the physical (and at times profound) sensations you experience as you're moving. Center around planning your breathing with your developments, for instance, or notice how the air or daylight feels on your skin. Adding this care component will assist you with breaking out of the pattern of negative contemplations that frequently go with overpowering pressure.

***Tip 5:* Associate with others**

There isn't anything more quieting than investing quality energy with another individual who causes you to have a solid sense of security and perception. Eye-to-eye cooperation sets off an outpouring of chemicals that checks the body's cautious "instinctive" reaction.

It's inclination's regular pressure reliever (if that wasn't already enough, it additionally helps fight off wretchedness and uneasiness). So make it a highlight interface consistently — and face-to-face — with loved ones.

Remember that individuals you converse with don't need to have the option to fix your pressure. All they need to do is be good listeners. What's more, make an effort not to let stresses over looking powerless or being a weight hold you back from opening up. Individuals who care about you will be complimented by your trust. It will only bolster your relationship.

Guidelines for forming relationships

- Contact a partner at work.
- Help another person by chipping in.
- Eat or espresso with a companion.
- Instruct a loved one to regularly check in with you.
- Call or email a close buddy.
- Take a stroll with an exercise pal.
- Set up a dinner date once a week.

- Meet new individuals by taking a class or joining a club.
- Trust in a pastorate part, educator, or sports mentor.
- Join a care group — either face-to-face or through an internet-based treatment stage.

Tip 6: Set Aside a Few Minutes for Entertainment only and Relaxation

Past an assume responsibility approach and an uplifting perspective, you can diminish pressure in your life by cutting out "personal" time. Try not to get so up to speed in the buzzing about of life that you neglect to deal with your necessities. Supporting yourself is a need, not an extravagance; You'll be better able to deal with the stresses of life if you make time for fun and relaxation regularly.

Put away recreation time; Include time for relaxation in your daily routine. Try not to permit different commitments to infringe. This is your opportunity to have some time off from all liabilities and re-energize your batteries.

Accomplish something you partake in each day. Make time for things you enjoy doing in your spare time, such as stargazing, playing the piano, or fixing your bike. Keep your comical inclination.

This incorporates the capacity to giggle at yourself. The demonstration of chuckling assists your body with battling pressure in various ways. Take up an unwinding practice. Unwinding procedures like yoga, reflection, and profound breathing initiate the body's unwinding reaction, a condition of serenity that is something contrary to the survival or preparation stress reaction. As you learn and rehearse these strategies, your feelings of anxiety will diminish and your psyche and body will become quiet and focused.

Tip 7: **Improve your Time Management**

A lot of stress can result from poor time management. At the point when you're extended excessively slightly and later than expected, it's difficult to keep cool-headed and centered.

Additionally, you'll be enticed to stay away from or cut back on every one of the solid things you ought to be doing to hold stress under tight restraints, such as mingling and getting sufficient rest. The good news is that you can find ways to improve your work-life balance.

Don't put in too much effort ; Try not to plan things one after the other or attempt to fit a lot into one day. Again and again, we underrate how long things will require.

Focus on errands; Cause a rundown of undertakings you need to do, and tackle them arranged by significance. Do the high-need things first. Assuming that you have something especially unsavory or distressing to do, get it over with right on time. The remainder of your day will be more charming.

Divide projects into manageable steps; If an enormous task appears to be overpowering, make a bit-by-bit plan. Instead of tackling everything at once, concentrate on one manageable step at a time.

Distribute authority; You can ask for help when you need it, and you can delegate tasks to others when appropriate. On the off chance that others can deal with the errand, why not let them? Relinquish the craving to control or supervise every last step. You'll relinquish superfluous stress simultaneously.

Tip 8: **Keep up with Offset with a Sound Way of Life**

Notwithstanding customary activity, there are other solid way of life decisions that can expand your protection from stress.

Eat a solid eating regimen. All around fed bodies are more ready to adapt to pressure, so be aware of what you eat.

Start your day off right with breakfast, and throughout the day, eat well-balanced, nutritious meals to keep your energy up and your mind clear.

Decrease caffeine and sugar. The mood and energy often return to normal after the brief "highs" that sugar and caffeine provide.

By lessening how much espresso, soda pops, chocolate, and sugar snacks are in your eating routine, you'll feel more and you'll rest better.

Stay away from liquor, cigarettes, and medications. Self-curing with liquor or medications might give a simple departure from stress, however the alleviation is not at all permanent. Try not to stay away from or cover the main thing; manage issues head-on and with an unmistakable brain.

Get sufficient rest. Satisfactory rest energizes your psyche, as well as your body. Feeling tired will expand your pressure since it might make you think nonsensically.

Tip 9: Figure Out How to Assuage Pressure at the Time

At the point when you're fatigued by your regular drive, trapped in a distressing gathering at work, or seared from one more contention with your companion, you want a method for dealing with your feelings of anxiety at present.

That is where fast pressure help comes in. Using your senses—what you see, hear, taste, and touch—or engaging in a soothing movement is the fastest way to reduce stress. By surveying a most loved photograph, smelling a particular fragrance, paying attention to a most loved piece of music, tasting a piece of gum, or embracing a pet, for instance, you can rapidly unwind and concentrate on yourself.

CONCLUSION

In conclusion, consuming excessive amounts of sugar can lead to weight gain, skin breakouts, type 2 diabetes, and an increased risk of various serious health conditions. It is important to limit sugar intake to under 10% of daily calories to maintain overall well-being.